CASETAKING
For the ENERGY PRACTITIONER

MELINDA H. CONNOR
D.D. Ph.D. AMP FAM

Other books by Melinda H. Connor

Ten daily needs
See auras
Accessing Truth: Emotion, Intuition and
Compassion (book and workbook)

Resonance Modulation: Biofield Basics

Advanced Body Reading

Casetaking for the Energy Practitioner

Professional Practice for the Energy
Healing Practitioner

CASETAKING
For the ENERGY PRACTITIONER

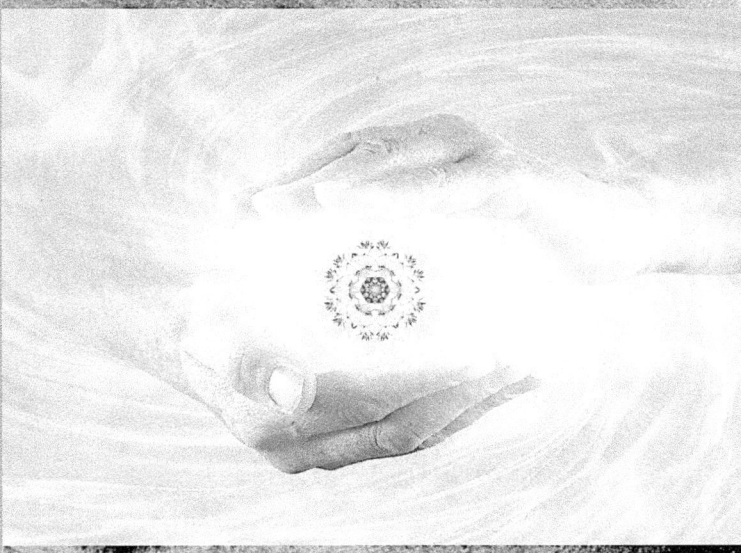

MELINDA H. CONNOR
D.D. Ph.D. AMP FAM

The material contained in this book has been written for
informational purposes and is not intended as a substitute for
medical advice, nor is it intended to diagnose, treat, cure,
or prevent disease. If you have a medical issue or illness,
consult a qualified physician.

Published by

ARNICA PRESS
www.ArnicaPress.com

THE DISCLAIMER
PLEASE READ BEFORE READING THE BOOK

The information presented in this book is educational in nature and is provided only as general information. You agree to assume and accept full responsibility for any and all risks associated with techniques and methods described in this book and agree to accept full and complete responsibility for applying what you may learn from reading this book. using any of the suggestions, approaches, the reading this book and using the information contained herein. By continuing to read this book, you agree to fully release, indemnify, hold harmless, the author and others associated with the publication of this book from any claim or liability and for any damage or injury of whatsoever kind or nature which you may incur arising at any time out of or in relation to your use of the information presented in this book. If any court of law rules that any part of this Disclaimer is invalid, the Disclaimer stands as if those parts were struck out.

BY CONTINUING TO READ THE BOOK
YOU AGREE TO THE DISCLAIMER

PLEASE ENJOY THE BOOK AND HAVE FUN!

To My Students,

May you dance in the rain, laugh with the wind, burn with passion, honor the earth and its people and love life to the fullest!

Blessings,

Melinda

ACKNOWLEDGMENTS

This book is the result of requests made by students over the last ten years. Thanks to each and every one of you for the beauty you have brought into my life. Berney, I am super grateful that you agreed to do the foreword. I have learned so much from our years of contact. You are ever the teacher and ever the wise one. Thank You!!!

Special thanks go to Dr. Kendra H. Gaines for her editorial wisdom through the various incarnations of this book. Kendra, you are a blessing in my life. Special thanks also go to Monica Heuser for her amazing eye for finding errors in the copy. Any errors in the book are mine alone.

A thank you filled with gratitude and much more piece of mind to Dr. Midge Murphy who keeps me straight in all things legal. To the team at Lulu Publishing, you are wonderful. Blessings Caitlin, you are the best daughter ever. To each and every person who has had a part in this book, thank you, thank you!!!

FOREWORD
BY BERNARD O. WILLIAMS, PH.D.

I f you have this book in your hands, chances are you are a practicing healer or are exploring the practice of healing. Herein Melinda Connor shares her methods of preparing a *"roadmap"* or plan for supporting a client's healing.

In this book, Melinda shares the lessons she has learned from studying and practicing many modes of healing work, herein laid out as principles for obtaining the information needed to understand who a client is and what is their spiritual journey. This books does not teach how to practice, for that you draw from your own training, and can also consult Melinda's other books.

Melinda holds a doctorate in psychology and her mother was a psychiatrist. In this discussion Melinda often emphasizes the character of healing work by contrast with psychotherapy or medical practice. *"Do not listen as a therapist. As a healer you are not a therapist. Instead listen as a friend."*

Melinda is one of those people who lives the passion in compassion. I first met Melinda at a meeting of the International Society for the Study of Subtle Energy and Energy Medicine. She had convened a session in collaboration with her colleagues Tom Firor and Michal Levin, exploring how to envision a common code of ethics across the wide range of healing practices. I remember one of the key points they made being the need for knowing when you don't know how to help, and the responsibility for referring a client to someone who might know better.

Now, more than a decade has passed since that forum, and Melinda is still advising that one of the key principles of working as an energy healer is knowing when and how to refer a client to another practitioner to help with aspects of a person's healing. Often the *"roadmap"* Melinda's method develops will include recommendations for other therapies, psychological and medical, to assist with the many layers in which energy blockages can be held.

Melinda also freely advises energy healers to pursue their own healing, especially if they are using their practice to try to heal themselves. As she says: *"If you are using your clients to make yourself feel whole, get therapy."*

Melinda provides examples of the myriad ways people can communicate their condition and processes of health or dis-ease, Melinda hyphenates this term, to emphasize the dynamics of health and illness. And she recommends giving much careful time to recording and understanding your case records. As she emphasizes: *every piece of introspective information that can be of value to the client should be included in the chart notes, Reminding clients of their prior flashes of insight can support their healing journey."*

Melinda is very frank about the potential of energy healing: *"You will need to record miracles in the record. Be sure to record those that the client has already experienced and those that come as part of the transformative process. Energy practitioners are involved in miracles. In a different century it might have been called magic. The transformations we support are only called miracles at this point in time because we do not yet have the science to explain what is happening.*" Melinda is also a pioneer in developing that science. She has conducted and participated in far reaching research on the character of healers and healing and has herself evolved new methods for exploring the dynamics of this magic.

We cannot expect to midwife miracles without sufficient care, and Melinda urges that we invest sufficient time to honor the importance and purpose of the practice: *"It can be argued that since in out current society 'time is money,' the case taking process is too long. I would counter that to fail to take comprehensive case information is a major ethical violation. The client deserves the best that you have in terms of skill, compassion and support, all given within appropriate boundaries and behaviors. Take the time in the beginning. It makes you more effective in the long term."*

The passion in Melinda's compassion is expressed in her core principles: *"The client is a sacred work of art, who is worthy of appreciation and gratitude. Create a space of kindness, compassion and truth."*

Berney Williams

Berney Williams is the President of Holos University Graduate Seminary and a Past President of the International Society for the Study of Subtle Energies and Energy Medicine (ISSSEEM). He has also served as the editor of *Subtle Energies and Energy Medicine*, the ISSSEEM journal.

TABLE OF CONTENTS

CHAPTER ONE ~ The Setting

CHAPTER TWO ~ The Steps in Case taking

CHAPTER THREE ~ Styles of Questions

CHAPTER FOUR ~ Language of the Client

CHAPTER FIVE ~ The Relationship Dynamic

CHAPTER SIX ~ The Process of Case Analysis

CHAPTER SEVEN ~ The Road Map/Plan of Action

CHAPTER EIGHT ~ Final Words

INTRODUCTION

CASE TAKING IS AN ART

Case taking is an art. It is not a science. Every case is different because every human is different. When you take information from a client you are being offered a gift that is deep and beautiful. Remember to stand in appreciation of the other person who has offered you this gift. This is the window into their world.

REMEMBER TO REFER!

Remember to refer the client if you are not the correct person to work with them. Know your legally defined scope of practice. No one is the correct healer for everyone. Do not allow financial considerations to lead you to make a tragic mistake. Do not fall in love with or seduce your client. Once they are your client, they will be your client for the rest of this lifetime. If your client looks tasty, refer. If you are using your clients to make yourself feel whole, get therapy.

DO NOT HURRY

Do not hurry. Give your client the gift of time. Time for them to form their thoughts. Time for them to breathe. Time for them to have the stressors in their lives fall away. Time for them to feel and become more real as a person.

LISTEN FULLY TO YOUR CLIENT

Listen fully to your client. It is possible even probable that no one has ever really listened to what your client has to say. Do not listen as a therapist. As a healer you are not a therapist. Instead listen as a friend. Listen without judgment.

Remember Gratitude!

Remember to have gratitude in your dialogues and in your heart as you speak with your client. Gratitude is one of the closest emotions to enlightenment and you will hear what a client has to say differently because you listen from this place.

Hold the space sacred

Hold the space of your case taking sacred. This is the physical space, emotional space, mental space and time/space. Keep the area clean. Keep the area as peace filled as possible. Keep the area imbued with grace.

Breathe Kindness

Breathe kindness into the area where you are working. Breathe it with every breath that you take in the space. Breathe it through you and let that kindness sink into your bones.

Let the client's truth be their own

Let the client's truth be their own. Truth is not relative. It is a real thing. Look to see if your client is standing/sitting in the light of truth as they speak. If they are standing in the light of truth, do not correct them, belittle them, tell them that their perception is incorrect and try to crowbar them into your format of the truth. Truth does not protect you or make you right, but it is a relief. Allow your client the relief of truth.

And in the last analysis all is just love. Remember that and do not judge.

CHAPTER ONE

THE SETTING

The setting of a case taking can support or hinder the process. It is important to support the client when the journey toward health and healing is likely to be arduous. Think carefully about the space you are creating. It is as much an internal space inside your self as it is an external space in which the client does their sharing.

PHYSICAL ENVIRONMENT

The physical setting for a case taking should be clean and comfortable with a minimum of external noise. If you are working with children, have an age-appropriate play box. If you are working with teenagers, have a separate space in which the parents may wait. If you are working with adults, have a space where they can speak without interruption. Be sure you have enough places for everyone to sit and options for how they sit. Some children talk more comfortably when they sit on the floor and play. Some adults do too.

In all of these cases have any chart materials, note taking material and forms that you need readily at hand. Be prepared with your chart materials prepped in advance. The client is not paying you to put your records together. The client is paying you to help them. Make sure that you have spare pens and other materials that you might need. It looks sloppy and is a reflection on the quality of your work when you are unprepared. If you use a tape recorder, check with the client to be sure they are comfortable with you taping the session. Many people are not comfortable with that process.

Be sure to remind the client to turn off their cell phone and other tech toys. Even better, if they are a high-profile client, have them take the battery out of the phone and if they brought one in to the session, their computer. Lots of people have access to the technology to dial into a cell phone or computer modem and listen to all that is going on around the phone. Be sure to turn your office phone down before your sessions and turn on your answering machine if you do not have administrative support or an answering service. This is respectful of the client. Turn on background music if you are in an area where someone might overhear confidential information. Better yet only take confidential information in a safe and protected setting! Sound travels. Be aware that you have an ethical and legal obligation to the client to protect their information.

THE SITUATION

I had a personal experience many years ago, where a practitioner was 10 minutes late starting with me, spent 10 minutes putting the chart together, paid no attention to the information which I was giving to them as they put the chart together and then they finished the session as if we had started on time by saying that they had to go to a meeting. They then charged for a full hour and did not offer to make up the time.

The Teaching

What might have been a better way to handle this situation? First, having the chart properly prepared. If you cannot, then wait until the session is finished and put the chart together after the client has left. You will have knowledge of the information you need for your charts. Ask the questions and take notes. Fill the information out later. Second, apologize for being late and arrange to make up the time or charge the client a reduced rate for that day. Third, if you have to leave early as well as being late offer to reschedule with the client. They may want to do a partial session but let them know up front the situation so that they can participate in the solution. Finally, you can still listen effectively to the client.

Internal Environment

The environment internal to the self is equally as important as a safe physical space. Good self-care is not just something that you work on as a practitioner. It is a job requirement. You must walk the talk and live your life from a place of balance and personal integrity. This translates to compassion toward the self.

Have a plan to do what nurtures you and do it each and every day. If you do not nurture yourself you cannot nurture a client. Eat properly. Get sufficient sleep the night before you will be in the office. Drink water throughout the day as you work. Take personal minute breaks. Plan them into your day. Learn how much transition time you need between clients to provide good quality healing support.

If you meditate, pray, take walks in the woods, exercise or do any of the other many things that you can do to nurture the self, be sure to schedule it into your week.

Understand how you maintain your internal balance. If you do not yet understand your own needs, start testing out and discovering what makes you happy, satisfied, and able to stand in the place of grace and compassion in the presence of another's pain. When you find the things that help you to hold that place, do them. Do them with discernment. For example: one does not take drugs, get involved with a client, or manipulate the people around them to make themselves happy and consider that because it makes them happy in the short term it is a justification for their actions. Rather, happiness comes from inside the self. Again, you must walk the talk as a healing practitioner. It is not enough to spout information; you must find the places of happiness, gratitude and compassion inside the self and nurture it. The answers are inside you.

CONFIDENTIALITY

Confidentiality is not a game. It is a matter of personal integrity and failure to maintain confidentially can result in a legal claim being filed against you. In our modern culture almost nothing is confidential. People whom you have never met can find out things about you that you had no idea were available to find. Correspondingly they can misinterpret the information which they find. In the healing room every word, action and thought of the client is confidential. Without written consent, nothing the client shares may leave the healing room except as required by law. Make sure you seek legal advice and know the federal and state laws regarding confidentiality. When you take case information it is important that the client cannot be overheard by someone. It is important that you do not share what you have been told except with a peer or supervisor and then only with written approval from the client and a sound reason for sharing the information.

Ask yourself, *why is this the case*? What is your understanding? What is your own answer? Words are often weapons in our culture. Information is a tool. It is a tool of power. It is a tool of control. It is a tool of dominance. It can be used for coercion. None of the information your client shares with you is to be used for those purposes. You will be receiving some of the most personal information a client can share. You will be making personal notes on the client's field and the images you see. You will be keeping records of the visits and the progress of the client. This information must be kept confidential and you are responsible for doing so.

To be successful, a healing situation must be in balance. The healing and the case taking must be done from a place of integrity and compassion. It is your healing room. You are the one responsible for maintaining the confidentiality of the client at all times. You must provide a space for the case taking where the client may speak freely and that is safe and confidential. If you cannot meet those requirements, do not take the case information. Wait and arrange for a confidential space.

THE SITUATION

One of the most common traps that new practitioners fall into is a mother, father, sister, brother, aunt, friend etc saying "I have permission for you to do a read on ..." Or they might say "Can't you just ask your higher self? I promise I won't share any information that you give me with anyone else."

THE TEACHING

What are some alternative solutions? Instead of doing the read, ask the person who asked for the read to be done to have their friend contact you. Give them your card. Share possible times that you would be available for a call. My belief is that you may not read a person without their verbal permission given directly to you or written permission given directly to you. If you cannot ask the client directly and outright, you do not have permission to read them. Ask the client and then stand by what the client says. Honor yourself and honor your client. Remember meticulous integrity!

CREATING A SAFE SPACE

O nce you have the physical space where you will be taking your client's case information, you must create the energetic space as well. For those of you who have been trained in skills like setting corners in a room, building containers, or building forms, it is wise to build a sacred space in which the client may share. This is not a religious space. A sacred space has an actual sound to it. The air hums. When you walk into the space, you will physically feel your body relax. When you experience the space, there may be a sense of timelessness to it. There may be a sense of joy that arises from being in the space.

For those of you who have never been trained in how to set an energetic space, I would suggest that you travel to a group of ancient trees. My first training in how to set sacred space was from a grove of oaks that was over a hundred years old. It was continued in later years by a group of two-thousand-year-old Redwoods in California. I used to love to sit at the edge of the forest and watch as visitors would approach the trees and suddenly fall silent, in awe and reverence and with a visceral recognition of the sacred quality of the space which the ancient trees had created.

Your clients deserve this space. You deserve to work in such a space. Learn how to create it and fill it with gratitude and joy.

EMERGENCY AND UNUSUAL ENVIRONMENTS

There will potentially be times in your career when you will be called upon to work on someone in less-than-optimal settings. It may be during your training when you can be expected to work in a larger group. It may be at a convention when there are people walking by your booth. It may be at a bike race with hundreds of people in the immediate area. Be careful of the questions that you ask in this setting. Speak quietly. Limit the information which you take to what you absolutely need to have to support the clients healing in integrity. It is not the place to go digging for the principle cause of someone's discomfort.

Appropriate questions might be:

- "What is the specific need that you would like to have addressed in this situation?"

- "In what way do you feel that I can support you best in this situation?"

- "Would you prefer hands on or hands off work in this setting?"

- "Would you prefer that I sit to the side and treat this as a distance setting?"

- "Would you prefer to sit in a chair rather than be on the table?"

Stay focused on your client and do not share information about earlier clients back and forth across tables with other practitioners while you work. Write your notes up where no one can see what you are writing. Keep your notes on your person or in a locked case. You cannot let them out of your physical control. It is unethical.

THE SITUATION

I was at a fair where a group of practitioners were sharing back and forth across tables about a client that they had all worked on over several months. It was very personal information. Though they never shared the client's name, it turned out that the client was standing at the next booth and heard all that was said. The client came over and the situation was made very public. The client was devastated!

THE TEACHING

A fair or public venue like a restaurant is never that place to share information on any client. If you need to share information with another practitioner AND you have the client's written permission, then move to a place where you cannot be physically overheard. Unless the situation is life threatening there is little information that cannot wait to be shared until the client's privacy can be protected. One of the very finest compliments that I can receive from a client is to have them say, "I have never felt safe enough to share that information with anyone before." I hope that each and every reader of this book will receive that compliment often in their career and hold the information with meticulous integrity.

CHAPTER TWO

THE STEPS IN CASE TAKING

C ase taking is a process and is often done over several sessions. There are a number of pieces of information that are valuable for a practitioner to develop so that they may support the client in their journey toward health.

ACUTE, CONSTITUTIONAL, RELAXATION, FIRST AID

O ne of the first assessments a practitioner needs to make is to determine the type of support the client will need. To begin the case taking process you will need to determine the answer to at least one of these questions:

- Is it to be long or short term?

- Is it to work with an acute issue?

- Is it to work with a chronic/constitutional issue?

- Is it that the client would just like a tune up or needs to relax?

- Is there some form of specific short-term support that the client needs?

To get the answers to these questions, you may have to ask something like:

- What has brought you here today?

- When do you feel this situation began?

- What kind of support would you like on your journey?

Most clients will be able to tell you why they came to see you. Most clients will be able to tell you if there is a specific issue that they would like to work with or on. Really listen to their response. How they phrase the answer can tell you a great deal about what they will need for support.

THE ROLE OF OBSERVATION

Once you have a starting point with the client, then you can begin your case taking process with observation.

You will need to answer the following questions through observation and dialogue:

1. How did the client walk into your office?
- Was it fast or slow?

- What was their movement pattern like?

- Did they have areas of holding in the body?

- Did they appear tentative, aggressive, tired, or were they experiencing any other specific emotion?

2. How did the client sit down?
- Were they awkward in any way?

- Were they stiff in any way?

- Were they emotionally expressive as they sat down?

- Did they take time to pick where to sit?

- Did they chatter or were they quiet?

3. As the client begins to provide you information:
- Were they emotional in any way?

- Were they sharing information in a particular style?

- Were they sharing information with depth?

- Were they sharing surface or story information?

- Did the client begin by telling you that you would or would not be able to help them?

- Did the client begin by telling you how to "fix" them?

- Is the issue they are sharing within your scope of practice or do you need to refer?

- Does the client have an adequate support system or do they need your help to develop resources?

The answers to all of these questions hold the potential to tell you a great deal about how to support your client. The answers will show you how deeply the client may be ready to work and may suggest how often they have shared the story of their experience. You may be able to determine how fully they are in contact with themselves and their issues.

Use observation as a tool. Notice what happens and do not judge what you see. Simply notate what you see and how the client responds. Information given at the beginning of the interview process will be useful throughout the time you support the client. Give the client an opportunity to teach you about who they are. Give the client the opportunity to share without you pressing a judgment upon them.

PRESENTING COMPLAINT, MEDICAL DIAGNOSIS AND THE FOCUS OF THE WORK

O nce you have notated your observations you need to isolate what the client's focus of the work will be. This would be similar, though not identical, to listing the presenting complaint. The presenting or chief complaint is the most frustrating, prevalent, or debilitating symptom(s) that the client is experiencing. The presenting complaint is the symptom the client usually came to a medical practitioner to address. The medical diagnosis is the listing of the disease or problem that is causing the symptoms that a client is experiencing.

The focus of the work is what the client decides that they would like to work on in their session with the healing practitioner. A healer can and should list a diagnosis made by a competent medical professional in their chart if it is available but a healer does not make a diagnosis. Often, the focus of the healing work and the medical diagnosis, have little in common. The diagnosis should be included as interesting information for the insight that it gives the practitioner on what kind of challenges that their client is facing. However, it is not the focus of the work. Nor is the client stating their presenting complaint providing movement toward a solution or resolution.

A client is either moving toward health or away from it. As a healer we support the client's movement toward health. We provide opportunities for stuck systems to become unstuck. We do not treat symptoms as this would be considered practicing medicine or psychology without a license which can result in criminal prosecution. Treating symptoms is the work of a competent medical or mental health professional.

So how do you determine the focus of the work? By listening to the languaging of the client around the situation in which they find themselves; by looking at the movement patterns of the client's body; and by looking at the biofield around the client. You can also determine focus by listening to the longing of the client's heart which they will eventually state if you give them room to do so. The information on the focus of the work is accumulated over time. So listen, observe, notate, study the person and their biofield, recognize patterns and reversals and give the client room to share what is in their heart.

The focus of the work can be different for clients with the same medical diagnosis. For example, if three clients have a medical diagnosis of diabetes, the focus of the work might be as follows:

For client one the focus of the work is developing the internal strength to be diet compliant.

This client is being supported in receiving energy sessions, learning meditation, breathwork, taking walks in the woods, practicing and allowing themselves to take 10 minutes a day to ground and do role playing and dialogue with the energy practitioner on how to hold boundaries. The practitioner is working with the client in conjunction with the client seeing a therapist (where they are focused on their family of origin issues) and a nutritionist who is helping to modify the client's diet to a more appropriate and supportive diet.

For client two the focus of the work is getting daily exercise. The client is receiving energy sessions focused on clearing sorrow and stuckness and learning meditations to support their work with their therapist. The practitioner is working with the client in conjunction with an exercise physiologist and a therapist. The exercise physiologist is tailoring the exercise regimen so that the client does not over-do and quit. The therapist is working with the client on self-esteem issues around being overweight and eating compulsively from boredom.

For client three the focus of the work is to help reduce the inflammation in the pancreas. The physician and the client made the decision together and asked that the energy practitioner work toward that goal in the energy session. The client is receiving energy sessions, learning qigong and keeping a daily journal to support mastering their negative thoughts. They came to the sessions knowing meditation but not caring about themselves as the result of many years of living with a physically abusive spouse. The practitioner is working with the client in conjunction with a therapist who specializes in trauma and abuse survivors, a martial arts master who is teaching the client how to protect themselves, and a physician who is working to rebalance the neurological and endocrine systems of the client.

Again, the medical diagnosis for each of these clients is diabetes but the focus of the energy work is different and specific to the individual. These three cases also illustrate how the energy practitioner, in contrast to the conventional practitioner, brings a separate set of tools to the table. Further, as is often the case when outside of an integrative clinic setting, the energy practitioner acts as a coordinator between the various health care professionals and supports the client on an ongoing, day to day basis in a way that the other health care providers do not have the time or the capacity to do.

MEDICAL HISTORY, SYMPTOMS AND MEDICATIONS

In addition to the medical diagnosis, a medical history and the client's description of their own symptoms is important to have as it gives shape to the organic and ongoing experience of the client. A comprehensive medical history can underline information that may have been left out in the information given to their physician but is important for the physician to know and for you to pass on to the physician. How the client describes their experience can illuminate their challenges. It will tell you a great deal about how the client uses language to express their difficulty and through the descriptions may underline areas where the client is stuck.

A list of all medications including over the counter, herbal and homeopathic medications should also be in the client record. While some countries have developed procedures so that medications are reviewed by a licensed pharmacist routinely, many countries still depend on the physician to do the medications review.

THE SITUATION

Joan came in to have a session with the specific focus of the session her experience that her mouth was always dry, and she always felt tired to the point of exhaustion. Joan was on three medications prescribed by her physicians and was taking two over the counter vitamin supplements and one over the counter herbal formula. In the process of dialogue, her medication list was recorded. A session was done teaching Joan to charge her body so that she was less tired in the short term and a teaching was done with an eye to helping Joan develop options for good self-care.

THE TEACHING

After the immediate session, the list of medications was reviewed by the energy practitioner, and three of the medications that Joan was taking, which were all prescribed by different physicians, all had dry mouth as a side effect. The energy practitioner then recommended that Joan talk with her physicians and her pharmacist so that alternatives could be found. Joan decided to speak with her pharmacist and the pharmacist then spoke with two of the physicians on her behalf. The two physicians put her on alternative medications and the issue of dry mouth was resolved.

In addition, the energy practitioner shared a teaching with Joan that her physicians also needed to know the entire list of over the counter and herbal supplements that she was taking. When the third physician learned about the herbal supplement, Joan was asked to change to an alternative because it was conflicting with her final medication.

Once that change was made, the issue of Joan's continuing exhaustion, while it had been improved by the energy work, was finally fully resolved. Questions asked of the client during the medical history, symptoms and medications section of the case taking need to include the client's physical experience of their body, the process in which they have been engaged to the point they began working with you, who else they have on their healing team, what has been done that has worked, what is still outstanding to work on or with and a full list of the medications they are taking.

A sample list of questions may include but not be limited to:
- Would you please tell me about what you feel is the state of your body at this time?

- Would you share with me what the process of your experience has been?

- What was the sequence of events that led up to this experience and the onset of your discomfort?

- How would you describe your current situation?

- What steps have you taken to resolve this process?

- What would you like to see resolved?

- What form would that resolution take in an ideal world?

- What medical and non-medical providers are you seeing at this time?

- How long have you been seeing each of these providers?

- Are you satisfied with each of these providers?

- May I please have contact information for all of these providers?

- What do you think are the underlying problems for you in this situation?

- May I please have a full list of the medications you are taking?

This includes over the counter, herbal and prescribed medications as well as food supplements, vitamins and homeopathic formulas.

Remember to take your time and really listen. Do not assume that you know what the client is going to say before they do even if you are a telepath. Listen to the words. Listen between the words. Listen to how the client pauses. Listen and identify when the client struggles to describe their experience. Listen and identify when the client tells you what their needs are in their current situation. Be careful not to tell the client that their experience is not so.

THE SITUATION

Charlene went to a medical practitioner for some assistance and shared that she was having regular back pain. The practitioner did a short physical exam and x-rays and on the second visit explained to Charlene that there was nothing wrong with her back and that she needed to see a therapist to work with her on stress related issues.

THE TEACHING

Charlene went to an energy practitioner when working with the therapist did not change her pain level after 3 months. Through listening and taking a careful case history, the energy practitioner discovered that Charlene sat in a chair that did not support her back for 6-8 hours each day. The energy practitioner referred her for an ergonomic assessment in addition to teaching her several qigong exercises and grounding exercises to help with her discomfort. An energy session was done to support moving the back into truth and relieving some of her current discomfort. This reduced her pain level to a 1-2 from a 6 as Charlene had subjectively measured it. As part of the ergonomic assessment Charlene's chair was changed as was her desk set-up. Further, it was discovered that the seat in her car was pushing one side of her hips forward. This was resolved with an insert placed on top of the seat and an adjustment to the seat position. Within a week Charlene had no further back discomfort.

It should be noted in the above case that the physician did what is required by the literature and could be done by the current standards of practice and in the time allowed by their managed care network. The therapist did assist Charlene with ongoing stressful life situations. Both provided good quality support. It just was not the support that was necessary to resolve the presenting issue.

FAMILY HISTORY

From a medical stand point taking a family history is focused on medical issues. Has anyone in the family had the same issue or difficulty? From an energy standpoint the family history is more focused on karmic issues. While the medical information may be relevant and can be included in the case taking, what is more important to learn are major family characteristics, types of behaviors that are common in the family, any patterned behaviors and episodes that include difficult interactions.

• What are the major themes within the family grouping?

• Is your client the black sheep?

• Is your client the identified patient?

• Is your client just like her mother or father?

• Is your client the only family member to be providing care for elderly parents?

• Is your client supported by family or providing the support to the family?

- When you dialogue with your client about the family, is there resistance to sharing information?

- Is there information shared in exhaustive detail?

- Is there a deliberate disconnection from family because of past traumas?

All of these types of questions can underline issues that can complicate the client's sense of self and ability to do self care. Further, the client may be involved in a repeating pattern of behavior or illness that is generational. So an energy practitioner takes family history about a client with this type of focus.

THE SITUATION

Henry felt that his world was crashing down on him even as he was happy in his job, had a solid family life and a stable income. All the family members were healthy. He did not feel the need for a therapist but felt the need for a greater spiritual connection that was not directly linked to religious belief.

THE TEACHING

The plan that Henry and his practitioner put together included exploring music, walking in different environments, finding activities that created a feeling of joy in Henry, creating a regular exercise plan (done through referral) and finding a specific creative outlet. Henry decided to take piano lessons and in a short time started doing monthly concerts at a home for the elderly. He stated that he felt he was finally "giving back to the community." In dialogue with the practitioner Henry discovered that his father had always wanted to 'give back' to the community but never had an opportunity to do so. Henry was very excited to discover that he was able to make a change in behavior from his family of origin.

CAUSATION AND DIS-EASE

It is very important to ask your client why they think that they developed the particular issue with which they are dealing. First ask, "What was the sequence of events that led up to your situation?" Most clients have a pretty solid understanding of the sequence of events and it can be super important to have that list. In my years of practice, I have had clients share exposure to nuclear material that they forgot to mention to their physician. I have had clients share accidents that happened the first time to them when they were children, and this occurrence was the seventh time for the same injury. All of this is very important information.

In addition to understanding why someone thinks that they developed their specific set of challenges, it can be important to focus on what they think is the underlying cause of their situation, dis-ease or dis-comfort. The sequence of events is different than the underlying cause. Ask both questions. Be sure to write down the answer to the question about the underlying cause as close to verbatim as possible. Remember, the language of the client in this situation can be a road map toward their resolving their challenges.

IDENTIFICATION
OF THE PATTERNED SYSTEM

During the case taking process, you will want to see if you can identify any patterned systems of holding in the client. This can be done by assessing the biofield, using a hand scan, or using visual assessment, extended sensing and dialogue. You may not be able to identify all of the patterned systems of holding without ongoing work, but the more information you can discern, the better.

Notate in the chart any places that are included in a patterned system and be sure to specify which patterned system is involved. You may find that this is most easily done on a drawing of the human body. Using a symbol and a number for each separate system can work effectively. For example: Using a star symbol for the particular pattern, then listing the position in that pattern and then listing the layer/chakra association can make the notation easy.

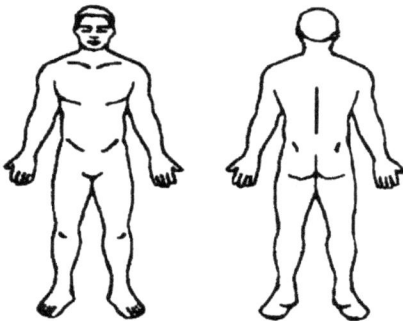

L – Layer

C = Chakra

* – pattern of flow in the field

*Physical report of bruising in balls of foot due to poor foot support when hiking.

(Referral to osteopath or podiatrist. Client choice.)

L1, left hip heat to 2 inches

*L1, right knee sorrow

L2, C3 cloudy and prickly

*L3, right hip lower

*L4, C4 thick and sticky

*L4 left side heat over shoulder to depth of 4 inches.

AREAS OF RESISTANCE
AND THEIR INTENSITY
~ STUCKNESS

When you are in the process of assessing areas of resistance to change or "stuckness" of your client, you will want to notice repetitive phrasing and descriptions, listings of what will not help them, listings of all the things that you will not be able to do to help them, all of the things which they have tried and have not worked and the level of verbal, body and emotional intensity as they share this information.

Notate for the record all of the information listed above. You may find that they have tried the same process over and over to get a change that has never been forthcoming. You may find that they have never tried the same things twice but did not do the work with the proper frequency or intensity necessary to produce change when they tried a particular mode of healing just once. You may find that they have exhausted every avenue open to them and have come to you for new answers and ideas. Each of these pieces of information will help you to set up the focus for the sessions and help you to support the client appropriately as they move forward.

IDENTIFICATION OF REVERSALS

In the questioning and dialogue process of a case taking, identifications of reversals can be a significant part of the discovery process. A reversal is where the client has a stated longing, for example, "I want to stop aching in every joint" and may have taken little or no action toward changing the situation. Sometimes the client will have taken some action, but it will have failed. It may fail because the client does not follow through on the action. It may fail because the client comes up with many excuses not to take the action. It may fail because of a level of resistance to change is greater than the determination of the client to make the change.

Finding areas of reversal and helping the client to adjust their goals into smaller pieces or finding better solutions that move the client forward with greater ease is important. Pay particular attention to sentences that begin with, "I really want to do XYZ but..." The client caught in a situation of reversal will often explain to you all of the reasons why a particular process will not work.

Reframing the process with something the client believes can and will support their process of change is necessary so that the work can be held in integrity. Teaching the client about internal communication can be a first step in helping the client create change in this area. So if possible, *write down the actual sentences the client uses.*

Once you have completed this part of the assessment process you can work more deeply with your information. Use meditation time to help you develop flashes of insight to support the client. Do research on the particular problem so that you may provide your client with the most up-to-date information available. Sit with the information until you have an understanding of the shape of the issues with which the client is dealing.

Remember, do not work outside of your legally defined scope of practice. Reversals may indicate a deeper psychological issue that needs to be handled by a licensed mental health care professional. You are expected to refer. You are not expected to be able to support all of the people in the world. Pick your clients using alignment with the truth and with your innate wisdom so that you properly support them and you do not betray them or yourself. Remember: no second victims! You do not make yourself ill in order to assist your clients.

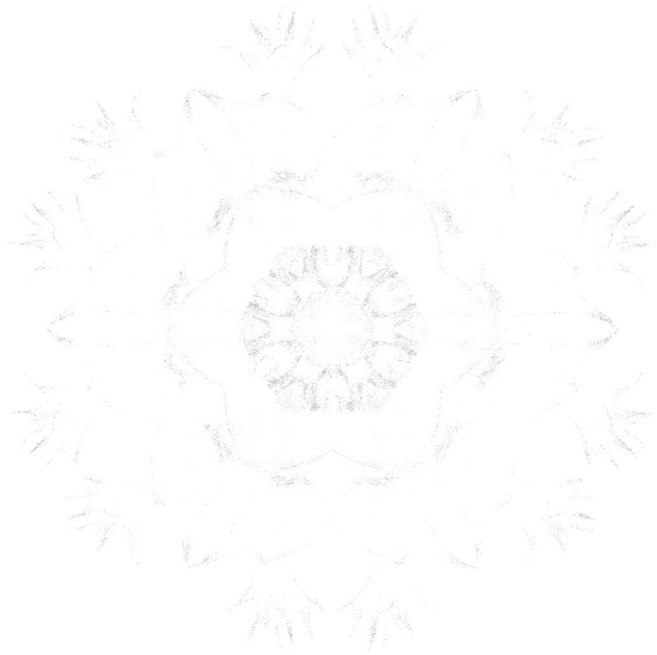

CHAPTER THREE

STYLES OF QUESTIONS

How you ask a question can be as important as the fact that you have asked the question. The selection of the type of question and the speed of the delivery of that question on top of an earlier question or how fast the question is asked are all part of the process. There are different styles of questioning. You will develop your own over time. Remember the client is not bad, wrong, stupid, an enemy or any other negative. All of your questions need to be asked using the following guidelines:

IS IT KIND?

Have you asked the question in such a way that it is kind? Most clients have had a difficult journey prior to coming to see you. Kindness is an important part of the dialogue process.

MORE THAN KIND, CAN YOU ASK THE QUESTION WITHOUT IMPLIED BLAME OR JUDGMENT?

You need to be aware of subtle language usage. Asking a question similar to "so what is screwed up today?" has a judgment associated with it. Keep your language very clean and precise. Resist using vernacular and catch phrases. You can use common language, simple sentence structure and smaller words if you wish. However, using words that have a quality of judgment should be avoided.

IS IT PHRASED CORRECTLY TO GET THE TYPE OF INFORMATION WHICH YOU NEED?

Think before you ask the questions or plan your questions prior to the client's visit so you ask the questions correctly to get exactly the information you need to support the client. Do not ask spurious questions. The client is spending money on you and you are spending your time and theirs. Ask questions to get the information you really need.

IS IT FOCUSED ON THE TASK AT HAND?

While asking questions that are unrelated may elicit useful information, most questions provide more information when they are asked in a logical sequence. People are more likely to remember important bits of information that can help you and help them if they are answering in a logical flow.

BE SURE THE QUESTION DOES NOT LEAD THE CLIENT TO A PARTICULAR ANSWER.

You need to ask the questions in such a way that the client gives you their answer, not your answer. An answer should not be implied in the question.

RAPID VS. THOUGHTFUL

When you are asking your questions, the speed with which you ask them will make a difference in how the client responds. Remember, you are not an attorney or a police officer so questions should not be asked aggressively. They can be asked at varying speeds. More routine questions can often be asked more rapidly so that you can move through the information you need and maximize both the client's and your time. More focused questions may require more thought or a more temperate delivery. Remember: Gentle and Kind!

PROBING

Probing questions allow you to search out relevant information or new information that may help the client. When you use probing questions you are on an information gathering journey. Phrase your questions so that they are more open ended and less specific as you begin to probe an issue and get more specific in your questions as you discover more information.

Examples of probing questions are:

• How do you think this situation has impacted your physical health?

• What did you observe about yourself at that time?

• Do you feel as if what is happening to you is linked to the family you grew up in?

• How did your children behave when they found out about XYZ?

Remember to use this type of question to fill out information about the client. Stick to the topic at hand. Only ask a question if it holds the potential to move the situation forward.

TARGETED

O nce you have a good sense of what the focus of the work is going to be for your client, if you still have questions, consider asking very targeted questions. This type of question will allow you to get very specific information. Do not ask aggressively. It is better generally to ask gently. Often when you ask a very targeted question, it can elicit an emotional response. Sometimes that response will be significant. A significant response should always be shared with the client's therapist or physician. It will provide them useful information as well.

Targeted questions should seek a particular piece of specific information. They need to be delivered in a conversational tone and in a matter-of-fact manner. Again, ask the question in a way that is kind. It builds rapport and trust with the client as you get the answers you need to help them as they journey.

Examples of targeted questions would be:
• How many times have you had this same type of injury?

• How often do you find that you cannot make yourself exercise?

• In what situations do you find that you cannot take a breath?

Remember to focus on important information and do not ask spurious questions. Keep the questions tight and on topic. Ask them in a way that is both kind and non-aggressive.

TRIGGERING OF THE DEFENSE

In the process of asking your questions, if you are asking them correctly, you will at some point trigger the client's defense. The point is not to ask questions to trigger the defense. That is the job of a therapist. However, the well explored history of a client dealing with a challenging situation will often trigger the client when they see clearly a piece of the work that has not been done or that edge them out of their comfort zone.

When you trigger the defense of the client you will need to deepen your connection to ground and reground the client. In many cases the client triggering will be the start of that day's energy work. Do not be afraid of triggering the defense but neither should you seek to trigger it deliberately in the case taking process. It is both wiser and more effective to have the client discover information through flashes of insight that bring them joy and excite them in the process of their journey than to trigger the defense.

In summary, you will want to follow the guidelines in asking your questions so that you can create a greater rapport with your client, establish trust and kindness between you, and allow for the creation of joy in the client's journey.

CHAPTER FOUR

LANGUAGE OF THE CLIENT

One of the most important parts of the case taking process is to pay attention to how the client expresses what is happening in their life, with their body and in their process, both emotional and spiritual. Thought has weight and charge.

Language has inherent power. It has information in the vocabulary the client uses and in the weight that the client places on each word. It will offer you insights into the perceptive process of the client and it will give you hints into their patterns of behavior.

In this process you will want to: *listen, observe, notate, analyze, verify and support.*

CLIENT BODY LANGUAGE

Observation of the client's body motion, style of movement, repetitive movements and points where they move to stillness can provide insight into holding patterns, areas of tension in the body, areas where the body is compressed or elongated, torsioned or shifted sideways. Remember you are an observer, and it is outside of your scope of practice to teach movement unless you have specific training in that area and have no legal restriction to do so. Nevertheless it is important for every practitioner to observe movement patterns. Also remember that the body is a chemi-electrical system. Electricity moves in the path of least resistance. Where there is no movement, there is resistance. Where the body is bent, the current will be in distortion.

THE SITUATION

Denise came to the session with the issue of acute neck and shoulder pain that had not been resolved with massage, chiropractic care or osteopathic care. She would have periods when it lessened because of the other things which she had tried but the problem would come back within a few days.

THE TEACHING

Her practitioner watched her as she entered the session and noticed that her shoulders were not level. The practitioner noticed that the shoulders were rolled inward and the upper chest was held very tightly. She also watched and noticed that Denise carried a very large handbag. The handbag was almost as wide as Denise's shoulders! When asked why she carried such a large bag, Denise replied that she had gotten in the habit when her children were small, and she had grown to like the convenience. The practitioner then asked her to put it on a scale and report back. The energy session was done to provide relaxation and release in the shoulder area with a focus on the full shoulder area. Denise called back the next day with the weight of the bag. Twelve pounds! The resolution: Getting a much lighter and smaller handbag.

Once again you will want to: *listen, observe, notate, analyze, verify and support.*

CLIENT'S LANGUAGE ABOUT THEIR BODY

It is not unusual for the client to use descriptive phrases as they dialogue with their practitioner. Many of those phrases are descriptive of what is happening in their biofield and often at a completely unconscious level.

Sample phrases might include:
- I am beside myself.

- I am ahead of myself.

- I am always behind.

- I am always trying to catch up.

- I have a cloud over my head.

- I feel like I am carrying a burden.

- I feel like my guts are spilling out.

- I am bottoming out.

- I am twisting in the wind.
- I cannot make a connection with anyone.

Many of the phrases describe exactly what is going on with the client. Check the body language of the client. For example, if the shoulders are compressed forward and the client states that they feel like they have a yoke around their neck, do be sure to check the charged fields in that area. If the client says they are walking through quicksand, be sure to check the area around the lower half of the legs. Often you will find distortion in the field structures.

COMPASSION OR SLANDER: THE ROLE OF JUDGMENT

As you listen to the language of the client, be very sure to note phrases where the client is telling themselves the following types of things:

- I always fail.

- I am never going to get healthier.

- No one can help me.

- No one can understand the pain that is my life.

- My relationships are never going to change.

- My job is toxic, but I cannot change jobs.

- I hate where I live but I know I will never move.

These are examples of negative phrases. The use of negative phrases in the client's language will often reinforce the belief that their situation cannot change. Stop them when you hear them use this type of phrasing. Help them to rephrase and keep reminding them to use the new phrases if ever you hear the old ones.

LEVEL OF INTROSPECTION

You will want to both use personal introspection as you observe the client and the introspective skills of your client to support them. There is great variety in the level of introspection of individuals. Some individuals have an acute understanding of how they function on a most visceral level. Most do not. However, every piece of introspective information that can be of value to the client should be included in the chart notes. Reminding clients of their prior flashes of insight can support their healing journey. In addition, it may again support the road map you are developing, with the goal of the client making the desired shift.

LEVEL OF SELF-OBSERVATION BY THE CLIENT

Clients will vary in their ability to recognize patterns, personal characteristics, and damaging behaviors. Self-observation is often linked to self-discovery. If given the opportunity, be sure to write down the client's specific observations. In particular, patterns and characteristic behaviors need to be noted. The information may then be used to trace patterns of holding within the body.

CLIENT PERFORMANCES AND PERFORMANCE ANXIETY

S ome clients will try to please you. They will tell you what they think you want to hear. Some clients will give you a performance when they hit areas of resistance. Do not judge. When you recognize that either of these is in progress, simply help the client shift back into truth. Help the client to refocus, relax and move forward in the work. Notate for the record the areas of resistance, and if possible map them back to specific areas of the body. Also notate when the client tries to please you. What is the area that you were focusing on at the time? Were they speaking about a memory? Were they speaking about a trauma? Were they emoting because they believe you want them to be dramatic or to cloud the issue you were discussing so that you will not focus on it? Remember, writing this information down will support the road map, the plan to support the movement toward health, that you are developing.

Once again you will want to *listen, observe, notate, analyze, verify and support.*

How well can you listen?

Listening is a skill. Listening requires patience. Listening and patience require practice. Practice with friends, family, business associates and everyone in between. Try to spend at least one conversation each day just listening to someone as you are developing your skills. Do not listen with half an ear. Do not listen from a place of distraction or boredom. Do not decide what the person means four words into each sentence. Do not judge. Just listen. Really listen to every word that the person says to you. In a short time you will start to have certain spoken sentences jump out at you. They will have significance. They too should be notated in a client's record.

There is a great deal of information that the client can provide to you if you take your time.

Remember to *listen, observe, notate, analyze, verify and support.*

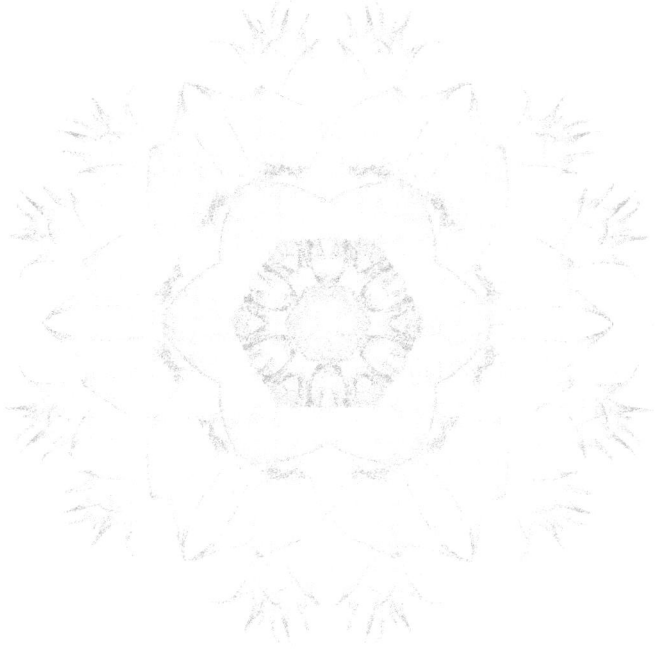

CHAPTER FIVE

THE RELATIONSHIP DYNAMICS

As you are taking the information for a particular case, you will need to have an awareness of the relationship dynamics between you and your client. There is always a power dynamic in any relationship and one of the core psychological concepts in ethics in helping professions is the power differential. Relationships that involve areas of vulnerability need to be carefully managed by the practitioner. A client who is trusting you to be a participant in their journey must be supported with the utmost integrity. Why? Many of the clients who come to visit you have seen lots and lots of other practitioners. An energy practitioner can be a person of last resort. You are the buck-stops-here person. You must, without exception, hold yourself to the highest standards of ethical behavior. To do so you must understand and never abuse the power dynamic between yourself and a client. Instead, you must use the power dynamic in support of the healing journey in which the client is engaged. Remember this includes appropriate boundaries and you are solely responsible for managing the power dynamic.

As you take the case information you must both be aware of and include the following information:

WHO HOLDS THE POWER?

- What does the client gain in this interaction?

- What does the practitioner gain in this interaction?

- What does the client lose in this interaction?

- What does the practitioner lose in this interaction?

- In what way does the client gain power or lose power when information is exchanged?

- In what way does the practitioner gain power or lose power when information is exchanged?

Acknowledging that there is an exchange of power is only the first step. You must also know where power is gained and where it is lost. There must be a level of balance in the healing relationship for it to progress. The practitioner will always carry more power overall and because of that power it is required that it be held with greater sensitivity, understanding, clearer boundaries and compassion. The client, however, carries the power of choice in the relationship. The choice to continue and deepen the work, the choice to make personal shifts and the ultimate choice to transform are all part of the client's power. So the balance between parties must be held with respect and compassionate understanding.

TRANSFERENCE, WHAT IS IT?

P art of the power dynamic in the practitioner – client relationship is what is called transference. Transference, both positive and negative, is at its core the movement of energy and imagery onto another person. My mother, who was a psychiatrist for over forty years, used to say, "There is no real healing without transference. It gives the person a way to see how the other person handles the situation and it gives them a way to heal themselves." After doing this work for so many years, I must agree with her.

Be sure to list the following in the record:
• When did transference occur?

• What form did the transference take?

• Was the transference positive or negative?

• How often is it happening in a session?

• How much charge is there behind it?

• What is the need behind the transference?

Again, this information is important as you build your road map. The episodes of transference will tell you what type of unresolved issues are present with this particular client. It will help you locate where there are subtle areas of holding in the body. It will help you facilitate the client's transformative process. Remember that this facilitation may include referral to a qualified therapist.

COUNTER TRANSFERENCE, WHAT, WHO ME?

J ust as the client may transfer positive or negative energy onto you, you may transfer positive or negative energy onto the client. Be aware when this happens and use therapy and supervision to maintain a good, appropriate, supportive relationship with your client. Be sure that you keep good boundaries.

SEXUALIZING THE TRANSFERENCE

O ne of the largest challenges in a healing relationship is sexualizing the transference. In essence, you would fall in love with your client in a romantic way. Energy practitioners are not like other practitioners. Once the person has been your client, that person is always your client.

You will never be in a romantic relationship with them during the current lifetime.
You must refer the client and sever the relationship if you cannot maintain appropriate boundaries.
You must go to therapy and you must work out your issues so that you have greater clarity in the future.

If during the case taking process you notice that you are sexually attracted to your client, do not wait. Refer to another practitioner immediately!

PABULUM FOR THE MASSES
AND STANDARD ANSWERS

O ne of the challenges that may face a young practitioner is the feeling of being overwhelmed. There are so many areas of which you need to have knowledge, and you cannot know everything. This is why you refer! You cannot know it all. People are too complex and there are too many places where people can have difficulty in their lives. That should not deter you from continuing study.

I have visited with many practitioners from various styles of energy work and received many sessions over the years. Try not to make the following mistakes as a practitioner:

1. The practitioner has not learned their craft.
It takes many years to build a competent practitioner. Taking two or three weekend workshops does not make you competent, no matter what wave forms or which styles of the work you have learned. Doing this work is a commitment to life-long skills building and learning about the many areas where life can make an impact upon us.

2. Gives standard answers when they have not developed sufficient extended sensing skills.
If you cannot sense what you need to so that you can do the work competently, do your skills drills until you can. This is called personal integrity and constitutes an honoring of your craft! You should at minimum prior to opening your healing practice be able to feel kinesthetically, hear, taste, and smell the fields that surround the body. Occasional vision, flashes of insight

and the ability to stand in truth, will, compassion, unconditional love, joy, your connection to your core self and your unique connection to the divine are also to be encouraged.

3. Uses blame when speaking to the client as an excuse for the client not moving forward in their healing.

The client does not fail. Only the practitioner fails. If you hold the space properly the client will move into it. If you do not have the training necessary for that client, refer! Blaming a client is also both projection and transference. Be sure to do your own good self management and get therapy and supervision on the client situation so that you do not repeat the error.

4. Makes believe that they can handle any case that comes to them.

Each and every human is a work of art. Each and every human runs their field with slight differences. As a practitioner you are not going to have the full range of frequencies or styles to work on every other human. Over time you will develop greater range but no one that I have ever met can meet everyone's needs.

5. Does not refer when the client is not making any progress.

It is not like you are going to run out of people who need your support. Go get some therapy and clean up your issues in this area. Then get a solid referral list together and use it. Be sure to write every referral into the record.

FEAR OF MIRACLES

You will need to record miracles in the record. Be sure to record those that the client has already experienced and those that come as part of the transformative process. Energy practitioners are involved with miracles. In a different century it might have been called magic. The transformations we support are only called miracles at this point in time because we do not yet have the science to explain what is happening. While we are developing the science (and it continues to get stronger; there are over 200 peer reviewed journal studies supporting the work just in English!) the practitioner in clinical practice must live in the current level of community understanding.

Do not fail to note something different in the records. What we do is different and needs proper, careful, record keeping. Do not fail to note miracles in the records. It is important to begin to understand our connection to the larger universe and our place in it. Even more important as the client begins their evolution, many miracles are possible. Miracles come in all shapes and sizes. When you note them in the record, you have them there to remind you and to remind the client when things are more difficult to transform and take longer to do so. *Remember that yesterday's magic is today's miracle and tomorrow's science.*

HOLDING THE FORM — WHY SHOULD WE?

As you are taking the case and watching the power dynamics in your relationship with your client, you must also hold appropriate boundaries. An example of this would be holding your clients to session time. If the client is late and did not call, end the session on time. Be sure to discuss why the client was late at the time it happens as it may provide insight into areas of resistance and help you build the road map.

Take advantage of the times when the client pushes the boundaries. Be sure to clarify and reset the boundary. Then be sure to dialogue on the specific meaning of whatever has happened. Again, it will give you information that is important to the transformational process. Remember there are physical, emotional, intellectual, spiritual, and energetic boundaries and you need to have a clear understanding of all types of boundaries when working with clients.

WHEN TO REFER

It is always a good time to refer! Be sure to notate all referrals in the record. Over the years I have found that in the first session information may come to light that supports a referral. It is wise to check out the people to whom you refer your clients.

Before I add a practitioner to my referral list I always go to them as a client for more than one session. It is important to me to be sure that everything will flow well for my clients and I need to understand the other practitioner well enough to be sure that it will be a good fit.

Many energy clients have had one failure after another, so assuring that the practitioner to whom you refer is competent, present, and will really meet the needs of the client, is important.

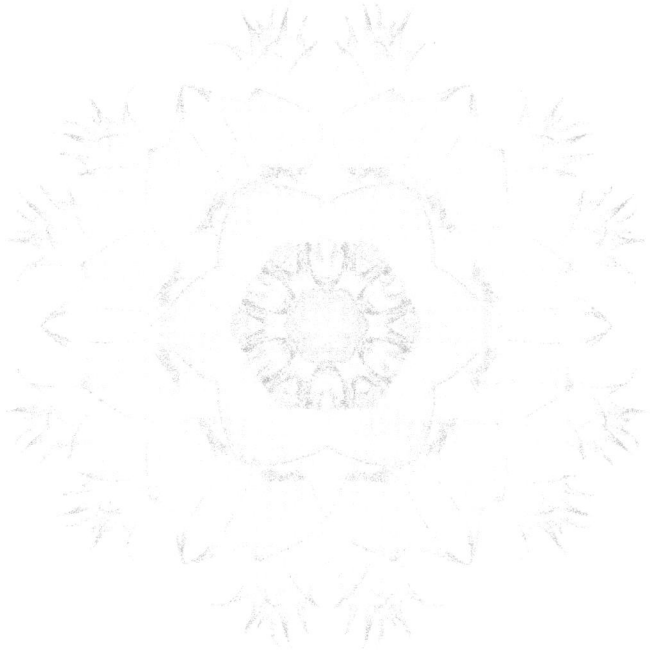

CHAPTER SIX

THE PROCESS
OF CASE ANALYSIS

Now that you have taken down a wealth of information, what is next? The next step is to sift through until you find the key information that will support the road map you are developing with the client. As you have moved through the case taking process you have been asked to note specific kinds and types of information. For example: If the client had one, what was the triggering episode of their discomfort? What are the symptoms and what does the client wish to focus on? What medication(s) are involved? How does the client describe their experience of their disease or discomfort? Forms in Appendix B will assist you in taking down much of the relevant information. (Be sure to check with a local attorney to discern if they meet legal standards for your area.)

SYNTHESIS

Once you have the information, you begin the process of synthesis with the goal of creating a road map for the client. During synthesis you will take each and every piece of information which you have been given and review it. Expect to take an hour or more for the review process. Be sure that you have all the information you need. Then try to understand the shape of that information. The shape of information means that you must answer the following questions:

- What is the core of the information you have received?

- Are you the correct person to support this client?

- What is the client's primary and secondary energetic defense?

- What is the underlying reason that the client developed this issue(s)?

- What has the client told you directly and indirectly about how to help them?

- What has the client told you about how their field is structured?

- What hasn't the client said which needs to be voiced?

- What will be the client's focus for the sessions?

- What other types of practitioners are needed to help this client?

DEFINING THE DEFENSE

Depending on the type of training program in which you are engaged, you may be taught a variety of models or theories about how the biofield is structured and how the body creates the biofield. For those of you who do not have training in this area, you may read my book, *Advanced Body Reading*. It includes detailed information on energetic defenses and areas of patterning. Those of you who have prior training in this area will want to pay careful attention to how the defense is interacting and holding the negative patterns of being in the body. Make note of this as you develop the road map.

WRITING UP YOUR OBSERVATIONS

Once you understand the shape of the information you have received, you can then begin to write the road map/plan of action for the client's support. Expect that every session that you plan will have things that will be adjusted in the now moment. Modify the road map/plan of action on a regular basis. Include what type of session, what protocols or techniques you will use and the reasons for that selection in each session plan. I find it useful to include specific references back to the case information so that the plan is clearly grounded in careful observation, client- specific information and listening.

RECOGNITION OF BODY DYNAMICS

R emember to pay special attention to areas of holding, patterning, and reversals. Include information within the record on how you will address each of these components. Remember to pay attention to places in the body where you have noted compression, elongation, etc. Finally, be sure to give particular focus to the areas the client described in body directed phrasing such as, "I am beside myself."

RECORD KEEPING

T he record keeping involved in the case taking process in the first few sessions does take time. Many of your clients have not been given the gift of time by their other practitioners since our current systems of care do not support that model. So that it does not become onerous, case taking can be done over a series of sessions. The information on a client can and should be added to continuously so that the client is properly supported. Session plans and the road map/plan of action may be continuously modified as new information is discovered and/or the client has new insights. I will often ask that a first session be two hours in length so that I may spend the first hour in case taking and still do an initial support session. The length of future session is always based on the needs of the client and their personal situation.

ETHICS AND COST

It can be argued that since in our current society "time is money," the case taking process is too long. I would counter that to fail to take comprehensive case information is a major ethical violation. The client deserves the best that you have in terms of skill, compassion and support, all given within appropriate boundaries and behaviors. Take the time in the beginning. It makes you more effective in the long term.

If financial considerations are an issue for the client, use a sliding scale. Only take a limited number of clients who cannot afford to pay your fees so that there is balance in that area of your life. Do take a certain number of clients who cannot afford to work with you otherwise, as an act of service to the community and to the earth.

For example: with very ill children I have a policy that if they are capable, they pay for their own support with drawings, poems, pretty rocks, a flower that they might have picked etc. If you feel called to donate all of this work to your clients, then you must have another job so that balance is maintained. I would note that I have found that when clients contribute at least something to the process they move toward health more quickly.

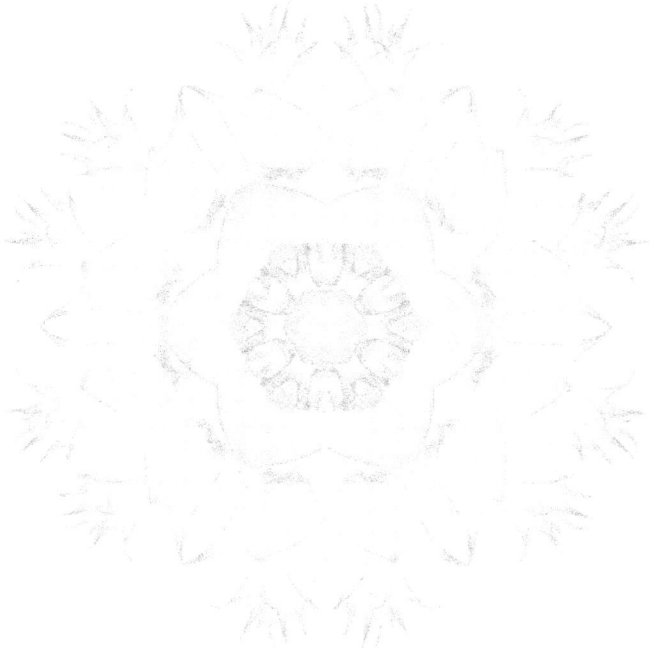

CHAPTER SEVEN

THE ROAD MAP ~ PLAN OF ACTION

The road map or plan of action for your client will be unique to each and every individual journey. It will outline logical steps to support the client. It must work within your personal scope of practice, your training and skill level and include all necessary referrals.

The goal of the plan at one level is to create oscillations in the biofield. Again, the body is a chemi-electrical system. If the electrical system is over-charged to the point the signal cannot get through the tissues properly, the chemi part cannot work correctly. Energy practitioner's work includes working with the electrical part of the system.

The goal of the plan at the next level is to aid the client in the return to their personal truth. This includes the truth of who they are, the truth of who they long to be and the truth of who they are becoming.

Logical Steps

The road map should be built around a series of logical steps. Each step needs to have a foundation in one of several possible areas: *physical structure of the body, emotional responses or defenses, negative and positive thoughts, lack of or deepening of spiritual connection, ability to cherish the self in an appropriate way, and the relationship the self has to others.* Remember, do not work outside your legally defined scope of practice or you could be subject to criminal prosecution for practicing medicine or psychology without a license.

For example: some energy practitioners are therapists. It is within their scope of practice as defined by law to do therapy on a client. Some practitioners are trained in yoga psychology, transpersonal or spiritual psychology, or some other psychological discipline. Again, they may do work with the client which is within their training.

An energy practitioner who is not a therapist does not do therapy on a client unless it is specifically within their personal scope of practice and they can legally do so.

For example, a non-licensed psychotherapist can practice therapy so long as he/she registers with the Colorado Department of Regulatory Agencies. The exploration an energy practitioner does with a client is a process of spiritual journey and is often called an Awakenings Dialogue (Lamb, 1999). It is a dialogue centered around the evolution of the spirit. It is not psychotherapy or analysis and should not be conducted in that manner.

-

Do Not Hurry

As you are developing your road map you will need to take your time. Plan on spending several hours, once you understand the shape of the case taking information, to develop the logical steps in the support process. Do not hurry. This person in front of you is a sacred work of art and needs to be treated with the same level of deep appreciation, gratitude and care.

Sit in Silence

For each and every client take a minimum of an hour's time and sit in silence with no agenda save that of receiving flashes of insight on how best to support the client. You cannot hurry this part of the process. You will need quiet where you will not be interrupted for the full hour. *Sit, breathe, and be.* And see what comes to you. Then notate and incorporate what is valuable from your time in silence. Use good quality discernment. Do not project. *Sit, breathe, and be.* And you will learn.

Writing up the Plan

The plan can be written in a list form, in paragraph form or in report form. You should, however, be able to read it when you get done and read it six years from now. I have sometimes worked with several generations of the same family and have found that reviewing those records can provide valuable insights into family line issues and trends.

Listed in Appendix B are several forms that can support the writing process. It is your choice how you write up the road map but the key elements need to be included. To that end, in Appendix C is a short form of the questions to consider and include.

USING THE PLAN

U sing the plan will help you help your client to move forward faster and with greater ease. That said, while using the plan is valuable, the analysis process and the subsequent clarity in your thoughts about the client is more valuable. Do not skimp. Over time you will develop greater skill in the case taking process and in the analysis process. However, in the beginning, take the time necessary to do the case taking and analysis properly. Your assessment skills will develop more rapidly, and you will provide greater service to your clients.

WHEN TO MODIFY THE ROAD MAP

M y road maps change every session for each and every client. This is because as a client moves through changes and develops new insights, the work deepens. As you are assessing the work your client has done that session you will need to sit with the question, "what's here now?" Modify the road map to meet the present moment.

CHAPTER EIGHT

FINAL WORDS

In Appendix C is a listing of the many questions included in the book in a shorter form which may be used until the practitioner is comfortable in the case taking process. Remember always that the case taking process begins with observation and good quality listening.
Do not think that you know what is going on. Check!
Do not assume you know what the client is feeling.
Fuse consciousness so that you really do know.

Remember in this process you will want to: *listen, observe, notate, analyze, verify and support.*

The client is a sacred work of art, who is worthy of appreciation and gratitude. Create a space of kindness, compassion and truth. Do not promise that which you cannot deliver. Be present to the client and always use appropriate boundaries.

HONOR YOUR CLIENT, HONOR YOURSELF, HONOR THE EARTH, AND HONOR THE DIVINE!

APPENDIX A: EXERCISES

1. FIND THE BODY CENTRIC LANGUAGE AND EXPLAIN HOW IT RELATES TO THE BIOFIELD.

Example A: "And then I when into work and I just could not seem to focus on anything. I mean I was totally spaced. I was out of this world."

Example B: "You would think that I could keep on top of things during the day. But no, I felt like I was always trying to catch up."

Example C: "I am just really, really down. I am always tired and I feel as if I have a cloud hanging over me."

2. WHAT IS THE PRIMARY DEFENSE?
(This exercise is based on a ten-layer defense model. For more information: Connor. M., "*Advanced Body Reading*")

Example A: "I keep telling him the way I do it is right! And he does not pay any attention to what I am saying. Nor does he do things the way I am telling him."

Example B: "You really want me to do that? Why would you want me to do that? I shouldn't have to do that…"
Example C: "You will do what I tell you. Go."

3. WHAT SHOULD THE FOCUS BE OF THESE SESSIONS?

Example A: "I really want to lose the weight, but I just cannot do the exercise with this ankle and everyone has tried everything and it just has not gotten better and I just ...."

Example B: "My blood sugar is all over the place. It drops 100 points in an hour. I want to start living a normal life and I just cannot seem to stay away from the fast food..."

Example C: "I cannot seem to stop crying. I am so tired, and I just do not know what to do. I talk to my daughter, and I feel a little better but between that and the hot flashes I just do not know what to do."

4. WHAT MAY BE PART OF THE PATTERNED SYSTEM?

Example A: "Well, I broke my toe and then about two weeks later I wrenched my knee and that was just getting better, and I got thrown off the back of the motorcycle and got a concussion."

Example B: "I keep injuring my ankle. I did some work to change how I move but it just gives way when I walk up stairs. It is the hardest to deal with when I am trying to get groceries up to my apartment and I have to watch the stairs..."

Example C: "Every time I shovel snow the small of my back goes out. I have a great chiropractor and a lovely MD but nothing they are doing seem to keep it stable. And I cannot go see them very often because I just cannot afford it. And if my back goes out, work is unbearable because I have to get up and down out of a chair that is too low again and again."

5. IS THERE TRANSFERENCE FROM THE CLIENT ON TO THE PRACTITIONER? (positive / negative)

Example A: "I always feel so much better after you work on me. Even when I do not have a new insight, I still feel better."

Example B: "You should have told me that it was going to work out that way. You are supposed to know everything."
Example C: "I have sent you a whole set of referrals. Isn't that great?"

6. IS THERE TRANSFERENCE FROM THE PRACTITIONER ON TO THE CLIENT? (positive / negative)

Example A: "It is just such a pleasure working with this client. They remind me of someone but I just cannot put my finger on who it is."

Example B: "They remind me of my father in the way they tip their head when they apologize."

Example C: "They are always so happy to be here. I do not feel happy today."

7. WHAT TYPES OF QUESTIONS WOULD BE GOOD TO USE?

Example A: "I really do not know why I came. My wife made the appointment."

Example B: "I just do not feel like I am making any progress with my life. I'm stuck."

Example C: "I am just so tired."

8. HOW WOULD YOU SAY THE FOLLOWING IN A WAY THAT IS KIND AND HOLDS NO JUDGMENT?

Example A: "That was a really silly thing to do."

Example B: "You should have paid more attention to the situation."

Example C: "Why can't you be more patient?"

APPENDIX B:
SAMPLE QUESTIONS AND TOPICS

1. How did the client walk into your office?
- Was it fast or slow?
- What was their movement pattern like?
- Did they have areas of holding in the body?
- Did they appear tentative, aggressive, tired, or were they experiencing any other specific emotion?

2. How did the client sit down?
- Were they awkward in any way?
- Were they stiff in any way?
- Were they emotionally expressive as they sat down?
- Did they take time to pick where to sit?
- Did they chatter or were they quiet?

3. As the client begins to provide you information:
- Were they emotional in any way?
- Were they sharing information in a particular style?
- Were they sharing information with depth?
- Were they sharing surface or story information?
- Did the client begin by telling you that you would or would not be able to help them?
- Did the client begin by telling you how to "fix" them?
- Is the issue they are sharing within your scope of practice or do you need to refer?
- Does the client have an adequate support system or do they need your help to develop resources?

- Is the work to be long or short term?
- Is it to work with an acute issue?
- Is it to work with a chronic/constitutional issue?
- Is it that the client would just like a tune up or needs to relax?
- Is there some form of specific short-term support that the client needs?

- What has brought you here today?
- How long do you feel that this situation has continued?
- What kind of support would you like on your journey?
- What is the specific need that you would like to have addressed in this situation?
- In what way do you feel that I can support you best in this situation?
- Would you please tell me about what you feel is the state of your body at this time?
- Would you share with me what the process of your experience has been?
- What was the sequence of events that lead up to this experience and the onset of your discomfort?

- How would you describe your current situation?
- What steps have you taken to resolve this process?
- What would you like to see resolved?
- What form would that resolution take in an ideal world?
- What medical and non-medical providers are you seeing at this time?

- How long have you been seeing each of these providers?
- Are you satisfied with each of these providers?

- May I please have contact information for all of these providers?
- What do you think are the underlying problems for you in this situation?
- May I please have a full list of the medications you are taking?

This includes over the counter, herbal and prescribed medications as well as food supplements, vitamins and homeopathic formulas.

- What are the major family characteristics?
- What types of behaviors that are common in the family?
- Are there any patterned behaviors and episodes that include difficult interactions?
- What was the sequence of events that led up to your situation?
- How do you think this situation has impacted your physical health?
- What did you observe about yourself at that time?
- Do you feel as if what is happening to you is linked to the family you grew up in?
- How many times have you had this same type of injury?
- How often do you find that you cannot make yourself exercise?
- In what situations do you find that you cannot take a breath?

- What is the primary defense of this client?
- What is the secondary defense of this client?
- Are they using judgment or slander phrases?

- What is the core of the information you have received?
- Are you the correct person to support this client?
- What is the underlying reason that the client developed this issue(s)?
- What has the client told you directly and indirectly about how to help them?
- What has the client told you about how their field is structured?
- What hasn't the client said that needs to be voiced?
- What other types of practitioners are needed to help this client?
- What is the focus of the work?
- Would you prefer hands on or hands off work in this setting?
- Would you prefer that I sit to the side and treat this as a distance setting?
- Would you prefer to sit in a chair rather than be on the table?

ABOUT THE AUTHOR

MELINDA H. CONNOR

B eginning her training as a child in the energy skills, she is the founder of Earthsongs Holistic Consulting & Executive Director of the International Journal of Healing & Caring. She is the lineage holder for the Resonance Modulation energy skills training program. Between Harvard, Wellesley, University of San Francisco, California Coast University, University of Arizona, American Military University and seminary programs, she holds three master's degrees and two doctorates.

Dr. Connor was trained in research as an NIH T-32 postdoctoral fellow in the Program in Integrative Medicine from the University of Arizona. Professor Connor, is the former chair of the board of directors for the National Alliance of Energy Practitioners and is also both nationally certified by NCCOEP and board certified by the American Alternative Medicine Association.

She is a lifetime fellow of the Royal Society of Medicine in the UK, professor emerita and former research director at Akamai University, and the author of ten books. Professor Connor has received both international awards from *CEO Today Magazine* and *Finance Monthly* and US recognition from the *California State Legislative Assembly*. Named a top research scientist by the World Qigong Congress and Marquis Who's

Who, she was recently bestowed with the prestigious title of Empowered Woman of the Year for 2024 by the International Association of Top Professionals (IAOTP). This recognition is a testament to her outstanding leadership, unwavering dedication, and unparalleled commitment to the industry.

WWW.DRMELINDAHCONNOR.COM
WWW.EARTHSONGS.COM
WWW.IJHC.ORG

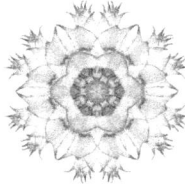

www.ingramcontent.com/pod-product-compliance
Lightning Source LLC
Chambersburg PA
CBHW071111210326
41519CB00020B/6265